The Art of Knife Play

A Guide to Safety, Consent & Introductory Techniques

The Progressive Kink Series

Sarah Newbold

PTC Publishing

This book is intended for mature audiences (18+). It contains content related to edge play, kink, and other adult themes. Reader discretion is advised.

when the blade hovers close,

it offers not pain but a breathless want,

a secret we can't keep.

this is the vow we forge in fire—

sharp with desire, deep in trust.

feel the steel against your skin,

taste the tension in every shallow breath:

don't stop, show me you care.

we live in the space between surrender and
command,

where every gasp becomes a plea,

and on that razor-thin line

we learn how fiercely we can hold each other

without ever letting go.

Disclaimer & Scope

Legal and Personal Responsibility

Welcome to this guide on knife play. If you're here, you're likely curious about the sensations, power dynamics, and intensity that come with it. This book focuses on external sensation play—no cutting, no blood play.

Before we get started, let's go over some important points about safety, responsibility, and legal considerations.

• **This Is Not Professional Advice** – This book is a resource for exploring knife play safely, but it is not a substitute for legal or medical advice. I'm not a lawyer or medical professional, so if you have legal questions or health concerns, please consult the relevant experts.

• **Know Your Local Laws** – Knife and BDSM regulations vary depending on where you live. It's important to check the laws in your area and make informed decisions.

• **Health Considerations** – If you or your partner have any physical or mental health conditions, speaking with a qualified professional beforehand can help ensure that your exploration is safe and comfortable for everyone involved.

No Blood, No Cutting

Knife play can take many forms, and different people define it in different ways. In this book, we're focusing exclusively on external sensation play—meaning no breaking the skin, no blood, and no cutting. If you're looking for information on more advanced forms of knife play that involve wounds or bloodletting, this isn't the right resource. My goal is to guide you through the psychological and sensory aspects of knife play, while prioritising safety and care.

Consent Comes First

Consent is essential at every stage—before, during, and after a scene. If at any point someone feels uncomfortable, everything stops. No exceptions. Consent must be informed, enthusiastic, and ongoing. If you or your partner are unable to communicate clearly—whether due to fear, substances, or any other reason—it's time to pause and check in. Knife play should only happen when all parties are fully present and actively consenting.

Understanding Risk

Even with external-only play, knives are still sharp, and accidents can happen—especially if someone moves unexpectedly. It's important to handle them with care and attention. This book provides guidance, but ultimately, how you choose to engage in knife play is your responsibility. Neither I nor anyone involved in publishing this book can be liable for how this information is used. Stay present, respect each other's boundaries, and remember—if consent or safety is ignored, it's no longer ethical knife play.

Inclusivity and Adaptability

Everyone comes to BDSM with different experiences. Factors like race, gender, disability, and cultural background can shape how you engage with play. I'll offer suggestions throughout this book to help make knife play more accessible, but ultimately, you know your needs best. Feel free to adapt what you learn here to fit your unique circumstances.

What to Expect

This book is designed to be practical, straightforward, and easy to follow. You'll find real-life examples, safety checklists, and best practices to help guide your exploration. Think of it as a conversation with a friend who has experience in the BDSM scene—take what feels right for you, and leave what doesn't.

On Land Never Ceded

This book was written on Dja Dja Wurrung land, where sovereignty was never ceded. I acknowledge the Dja Dja Wurrung people as the Traditional Owners of this land and honour their ongoing connection to Country, as well as their strength, resistance, and resilience.

The systems we live and work within are shaped by colonial histories and ongoing injustices. Decolonisation is not just an idea—it's an active responsibility. As part of this acknowledgment, I commit to:

• Listening and Learning – Centering Indigenous voices, supporting Indigenous-led initiatives, and incorporating cultural knowledge with care and respect.

• Action for Sovereignty – Advocating for policies that uphold Indigenous land rights, self-determination, and justice.

• Financial Commitment – Contributing 2% of this book's proceeds to Indigenous organisations dedicated to justice and healing for First Nations communities.

Acknowledgment alone is not enough, but it is an important step in continuing the work of truth, respect, and meaningful action.

Chapter 1
What is Knife Play?

When people hear *knife play*, they often imagine something extreme or dangerous. In reality, knife play spans a wide range of kink experiences. Some enjoy light, sensory contact with the dull edge of a blade. Others explore fear-based scenarios using a sharpened knife. While knife play carries higher risks than many other kinks, it can be managed safely with planning, communication, care, and trust.

This chapter explores what knife play is, why it's considered "edge play," and why some people are drawn to it. We'll also briefly touch on cutting and blood play—though this book does not provide instructions for those practices.

1. Knife Play as Edge Play in BDSM

1.1 Understanding Edge Play

In kink, edge play refers to activities seen as more intense or riskier than common kinks. Examples include breath play, fire play, and certain types of impact play. Knife play falls under this category because of its potential for (lethal) injury and psychological intensity.

For many, the perceived risk is part of the appeal. Knife play creates strong physical sensations alongside emotional and mental responses. Fear heightens these effects. Because mistakes can have serious consequences, risk management is essential. Knife play is an advanced kink activity that requires clear communication and proper technique.

1.2 Degrees of Intensity

Not all knife play is extreme. Some enjoy the cool, metal-on-skin sensation without fear. Others explore intense scenarios, like a blade held near a partner's throat in a consensual fear scene. There's a broad spectrum between these approaches. What matters most is that all participants are informed, comfortable, and able to consent to the level of intensity they engage in.

2. Knife Play as Sensory Play

2.1 Cool Metal and Precise Sensations

Knives appeal to some people purely for how they feel. A blade's smooth steel creates a distinct sensation. Unlike paddles or floggers, the dull side of a blade can glide across the skin, cool and sharp, heightening sensitivity.

For some, knife play is just about sensation — no fear, no power exchange, just an exploration of temperature, texture, and heightened awareness. This form of play can be meditative, intimate, or even playful.

2.2 The Role of Psychological Tension

Even in a light, sensory-focused scene, the presence of a knife can create psychological tension. That quiet awareness — knowing a blade is close but being used with care — can trigger an adrenaline rush, even when risk is minimal.

When trust is strong, this controlled tension deepens the experience. It transforms simple touch into something more intense.

3. Power Dynamics: Optional, Not Required

3.1 Knife Play and Power Exchange

Some incorporate knife play into power exchange dynamics. A top holds the knife, while the **bottom** experiences its effects. The top may use the blade to guide movement, enhance control, or create suspense. In fear-based play, the bottom's excitement may come from the tension of the moment, trusting the top's skill and restraint.

3.2 Equal-Partners Approach

Not all knife play involves a power dynamic. Some partners take turns tracing the blade on each other's skin. Without a hierarchy, the focus is on curiosity and sensation rather than control.

Knife play can be anything—a tool for power dynamics, a form of sensory play, or a mix of both.

4. Non-Penetrative vs. Cutting and Blood Play

4.1 External-Only Knife Play

This book focuses on external-only knife play, meaning the blade is used without breaking the skin —sliding, tracing, or applying light pressure. The goal is to create sensation and psychological intensity without harm.

Even though this book does not cover cutting or blood play, all knife play participants should have basic first aid knowledge, a well-stocked first aid kit, and a plan for handling accidents. Any time sharp objects are involved, preparation is key.

4.2 Cutting and Blood Play: A Brief Overview

Some kink practitioners incorporate cutting or blood play into their scenes. This requires much higher skill, including sterility, wound care, and an understanding of bloodletting's effects.

Because this play carries significantly more risk, it falls outside this book's scope. If you're interested, seek out advanced resources and mentorship from experienced practitioners.

5. Why People Enjoy Knife Play

5.1 Adrenaline and Suspense

A knife introduces a unique level of tension. The awareness of a sharp object near the skin triggers an adrenaline rush, making every touch more intense.

5.2 Heightened Body Awareness

Knife play encourages full-body awareness. The precise touch of metal is more deliberate than many other kink tools, making every sensation stand out. Some people find this grounding or even meditative.

5.3 Emotional Intimacy

Any activity involving trust deepens intimacy. The bottom entrusts their safety to the top. The top takes responsibility for control and precision. A successful knife scene strengthens connection and communication.

6. Risk and Reward

6.1 Main Risks

- **Accidental Cuts** – Even with care, knives are sharp. Unexpected movements can cause injury and potentially death.

- **Emotional Triggers** – Past trauma or fear responses may surface.

- **Relationship Stress** – Miscommunication or an unplanned outcome can strain trust.

6.2 Potential Rewards

- **Enhanced Trust** – A well-executed knife scene strengthens confidence in your partner.

- **Unique Sensation** – Metal against skin provides a distinct experience.

- **Psychological Depth** – The tension adds an emotional and mental layer to play.

7. Safety and Consent: A Preview

Before going further, here are three key safety principles:

1 Clear, Ongoing Consent – Check in regularly. Stop immediately if someone feels uncertain.

2 Communication – Discuss limits, preferred areas, and the type of blade being used.

3 Skill Building – Practice handling techniques before using a blade on a partner.

We'll cover negotiation, safety, and technical skills in later chapters. For now, remember: knives demand **intention, awareness, and respect**.

8. Final Thoughts

Knife play isn't one-size-fits-all. Some find it thrilling, others don't—and both are valid. The key is approaching it with **care, clear boundaries, and a balance of risk and pleasure**.

Next, we'll break down the **practical aspects of knife play**—covering technique, safety measures, and how to ensure every experience is both thrilling and responsible.

Chapter 2
Consent & Safety

2.1 Introduction: Why Safety Matters

Safety is often the first thing people worry about when they hear the term "knife play," and for good reason. Knives can stir up strong and often opposing emotions. There can be a tension between excitement, fear, arousal and playfulness.

When you understand how to negotiate boundaries, handle knives correctly, and watch out for each other's emotional well-being, you can transform what might seem like a daunting activity into something thrilling and deeply connective.

Many people are drawn to knife play because it offers a blend of physical sensation and psychological intensity that's hard to replicate with other forms of kink. A blade can feel cool, precise, and—frankly—a bit dangerous. For some, that sense of danger is part of the appeal, and the adrenaline spike it can bring is unlike anything else. Yet beneath that excitement lies an important truth: real knives can cause real harm if misused.

This chapter will explore ways to keep the experience consensual, enjoyable, and mindful of everyone's limits, ensuring that the trust you build in these scenes isn't broken by unintended mishaps.

2.2 Consent: Clarity, Enthusiasm, and the Freedom to Change Your Mind

Consent isn't just a formality to tick off before you start—think of it more as an ongoing conversation between you and your partner.

It's vital for both people to be on the same page about what might happen. That means detailing the types of blades, the level of pressure, and any forms of play you're not comfortable with, such as fear play or highly restrictive bondage combined with knives. You also need genuine enthusiasm—no one should feel coerced or talk themselves into it just to please the other. And remember, consent isn't locked in. If halfway through you find that a certain movement or sensation feels overwhelming, you have every right to pause or stop without being judged or pressured to continue.

Knife play is meant to be a shared experience rooted in trust and open communication, and that trust relies on both partners having the freedom to change their minds.

2.3 Negotiation Before Play

Before introducing a knife into your BDSM scene, it helps to have a frank discussion about what each partner wants, expects, and fears. This might involve talking about which parts of the body are off-limits (some people are comfortable with the blade near their torso but prefer it kept away from their neck), how long the scene might last, and the overall mood— do you want something slow and sensual or a more intense, edgy vibe? Think of negotiation as a way to paint a picture of your ideal scene so the other person can step into that vision with full awareness.

2.4 Knife Play Doesn't Have to Break the Skin

One of the biggest misconceptions about knife play is that it always involves actual cutting or drawing blood. In fact, many people find knife play enticing precisely because it can remain a purely external, psychological thrill. Picture the sensation of a blade trailing along your back or the inner part of your arm: it's a unique blend of ticklish awareness and the mildest hint of potential danger. That feeling alone can be enough to push the adrenaline button without making actual cuts. Some folks liken it to the gentle scrape of an ice cube, except with a different emotional charge tied to the blade's cultural associations of danger or taboo.

There's absolutely no requirement that you escalate to cutting. Some people do enjoy blood play, but that territory involves more advanced skills, strict hygiene protocols, and a high level of trust. If you're curious about the idea of drawing blood, you'll need far more specialised information and possibly a mentor who knows the ropes (and the scalpels). But for now, remember that a simple brush of steel against skin can be incredibly powerful in its own right.

2.5 Psychological Safety: Watching for Emotional Signals

While physical risk is often top of mind, emotional or psychological safety is just as crucial. A blade, even if used gently, can trigger strong reactions that catch people by surprise. That's why the top in a knife-play scene should pay close attention to the bottom's reactions, not just physically but emotionally. Are they breathing evenly, or has their breathing become strained or shallow? Do they look relaxed and engaged, or are they zoning out or trembling? If they seem suddenly quiet or tense, it could be a sign of fear, discomfort, or a flashback to a past experience.

A friend of mine once tried knife play without fully discussing her history of self-harm with her partner. Partway through the scene, she was hit by a surge of anxiety she didn't anticipate, and it nearly derailed the entire evening. The takeaway: emotional triggers aren't always obvious until you hit them. Regular "How are you feeling?" check-ins during the scene can help you catch any issues early. And if something feels off, it's better to pause, breathe, and talk it through. No physical thrill is worth pushing someone into an emotional crisis.

2.6 Knowing the Difference Between Knife Play and Abuse

When done ethically, knife play should never feel like an assault. Consent is the dividing line between a trusting, collaborative scene and an abusive situation. If one person forces the other past agreed limits, ignores safe words, or makes light of their partner's emotional distress, that's not consensual kink—it's abusive. True BDSM, at its best, involves empathy and respect, even when the activities appear edgy or extreme to an outside observer.

It's useful to set a clear safe word (like "Red" or "Banana"—anything easy to remember) that instantly signals "Stop everything right now." The top has to be ready to stop on a dime if the bottom uses that word. You can also agree on a separate safe word or code that means "Slow down" or "I'm getting close to my limit." That extra nuance can help you adjust a scene rather than end it prematurely. But if you use a stop word and your partner keeps going, that's no longer a kink scene; it's violation of your consent.

2.7 Physical Safety: Knife Care and Play Space

Physical safety starts with taking care of your tools and your environment. A poorly maintained knife can create unpredictable hazards, whether it's chipped edges or hidden rust spots that might lead to infection if the skin is accidentally broken. Keeping blades sharp, oddly enough, can actually be safer than using a dull one, because a dull blade is more likely to slip or snag. It's also wise to play in a well-lit area, free of clutter or tripping hazards, so you're not jostled unexpectedly mid-scene.

If you're new to knife play, consider practising on inanimate objects first. Some people like to hone their technique by cutting fruit or lightly tracing shapes on a cushion. It might sound silly, but it builds your confidence and muscle memory before you move on to live human skin. And don't forget to keep a basic first-aid kit within easy reach—just in case something goes wrong. Accidents can happen, and it's better to be prepared than caught off guard.

2.8 Safe Words and Non-Verbal Signals

Safe words are critical in BDSM for letting your partner know exactly where you stand, especially if you find yourself overwhelmed or nearing your threshold. But knife play sometimes involves scenarios where speech might be difficult—whether because of fear, a gag, or just the intensity of the moment. In those cases, a non-verbal signal can be a lifesaver. Some couples agree on a series of taps on the bed, a hand squeeze, or dropping a certain object to communicate "I've reached my limit."

Whatever system you choose, make sure it's clearly understood by both parties and easy to do in a moment of panic. Part of the negotiation phase might involve practising the signal once or twice so there's no confusion during the real scene. It's a small step that can make a big difference in feeling secure enough to let yourself enjoy the knife play.

2.9 Aftercare: Coming Back to Baseline

Knife play can stir up a swirl of emotions and sensations. Once the scene is over, it's essential to take some time to come down from the adrenaline high and reconnect. Aftercare often includes snuggling or a comforting conversation where both partners can process how they felt. If the bottom has any minor marks or scratches, cleaning them and applying antiseptic can also be part of the cool-down routine.

Interestingly, many people who enjoy knife play say that the emotional bond they experience in the aftermath is even stronger than in other forms of BDSM. There's something about the controlled risk of a blade that heightens the trust dynamic. By offering gentle reassurance, warmth, and acknowledgement of what you both just experienced, you reinforce that sense of trust and keep it from dissolving the moment the scene ends.

2.10 Conclusion: Building a Strong Foundation

Approaching knife play responsibly involves more than just picking up a blade. It's about crafting an environment where both partners can explore heightened sensations without losing sight of each other's well-being. The conversations you have beforehand, the attention you pay to emotional signals, the care you take in handling the knife, and the support you offer afterwards all weave together to create a truly memorable experience.

If you follow these guidelines—respecting consent, safeguarding physical and emotional health, and offering genuine aftercare—you'll find that knife play can become a uniquely powerful way to connect. The next chapter will delve into the nuts and bolts of handling a knife with precision, offering tips and techniques for those ready to take a hands-on approach to this exciting form of kink.

Chapter 3
Tools of the Trade

When people think of "knife play," they often picture scenes filled with overly large hunting knives or theatrical blades straight from a horror film. In truth, consensual, non-penetrative knife play is typically more about having a tool that feels comfortable, glides smoothly along the skin, and remains predictable throughout. Even though we're dealing with external sensation rather than cutting, proper knife care and smart selection can make all the difference in ensuring scenes feel safe as well as exciting.

A key point to remember is that a knife doesn't need to be huge or menacing to deliver the psychological or tactile thrill many seek. In fact, an excessively big or unwieldy blade might make it harder to perform the gentle touches or detailed tracing that characterises many people's first explorations into knife play. If you start with a tool that's manageable and easy to control, you'll likely have a more positive experience—one that emphasises skill and consent rather than grappling with a blade that feels cumbersome.

3.1 Why the Right Knife Matters

Choosing the right knife directly influences both the sensations you can create and your overall confidence during play. Some people are drawn to heavier blades for the dramatic effect they can offer, but it's worth thinking carefully about your ability to handle that extra weight. A smaller or lighter blade often allows for more precision, letting you explore subtle changes in pressure or speed without worrying that the blade might slip out of your hand.

Comfort in your grip is equally important. A handle that's too large or poorly designed can lead to fatigue or accidental slips, which is the last thing you want during a scene. It's not just about how a knife looks; it's about how it feels in your hand. At its core, knife play is meant to add a layer of controlled intensity to a BDSM scene, and that control relies on having a tool that behaves predictably under your guidance.

3.2 The Anatomy of a Knife

Although the aim here isn't cutting, it's still a good idea to understand the basic components of a knife.

You have the blade, which can be plain or serrated, the spine, which is the unsharpened edge opposite the cutting edge, the tip, and the handle. Some knives include a bolster or guard between the blade and the handle, which adds extra security against slipping.

The tip is often the riskiest part to handle, especially if you plan on using it for delicate, pinpoint sensations. Even slight misalignment in your grip could result in an unintended scratch or shallow nick. Familiarising yourself with these elements boosts your confidence and helps prevent unwanted surprises, making the experience more pleasurable for everyone.

3.3 Different Knife Styles for External Play

Paring Knives

A paring knife is typically three to four inches long and is an excellent choice for those looking for a lightweight, easy-to-control tool. While it might not have the visual drama of a larger blade, it excels in precision, allowing you to trace patterns or lightly graze the skin with minimal risk of accidentally dragging too much weight. Many people find it a natural starting point because it provides good finesse without feeling intimidating.

Utility Knives

If you prefer a step up from a paring knife, a utility knife — often four to six inches long—offers a balance between reach and control. Its longer blade can produce a more noticeable sensation on the skin, and some people enjoy the psychological feeling of wielding a knife that's a touch bigger. At the same time, it remains manoeuvrable enough for gentle strokes or firmer, more intense contact when you want to vary the experience.

Folding Knives

Folding knives come in a range of sizes, from very compact to medium length. Their main advantage lies in being discreet and portable, making them appealing for those who prefer a smaller kit or need to store the knife quietly. However, always check that the lock mechanism is sturdy. A weak or worn-out lock could fail mid-scene, which can be dangerous. If you choose a folding knife, invest in one from a reliable manufacturer to reduce the risk of mechanical failures.

Fixed-Blade Knives

Fixed-blade knives, which can include small hunting knives, have a blade permanently attached to the handle, meaning they have no moving parts to worry about. They're often sturdier and can offer a striking aesthetic that some find appealing. However, the weight and size of certain fixed-blade models can make them harder to control if you prefer a softer, more detailed style of play. If you do lean towards a larger fixed blade, be sure you feel fully comfortable with its balance and heft before bringing it near a partner's skin.

Decorative or Theatrical Knives

Some knives are made primarily for show and might feature ornate designs or dramatic shapes. While they can be visually impressive, quality and durability aren't always the top priorities in their construction. A decorative knife that snaps or cracks mid-scene poses a real risk. If you're drawn to an eye-catching piece, ensure it's well-made and can handle the movements of knife play without falling apart at the first sign of pressure.

3.4 Sharpness: Balancing Myths and Realities

A common question is whether a knife should be extremely sharp, moderately sharp, or quite dull. A dull blade might appear safer because it's less likely to slice someone by accident, but it can also snag on the skin, leading to unpredictable abrasions. A blade that's too sharp demands significant skill and concentration, as even a minor slip could cause a cut. Many people find a moderately sharp edge strikes the best compromise: smooth enough for controlled gliding without being razor-like. Ultimately, the right level of sharpness will depend on your skill, your partner's comfort, and the kind of sensations you wish to create.

. . .

3.5 Handling, Grip, and Comfort

The way a knife feels in your hand underpins every movement you'll make. If the handle is too big, too small, or oddly shaped, you might struggle to maintain a steady grip. Some knives are balanced so that the blade carries more weight, while others centre their weight around the handle. Consider running the flat side or spine of the knife along your own arm to gauge how easily you can keep a consistent line without undue strain. If the knife keeps wobbling, or if your wrist tires quickly, it may not be the ideal blade for your style of play.

3.6 Materials, Maintenance, and Overall Care

Knife materials vary, with stainless steel being a popular, rust-resistant option and carbon steel prized by those who prefer a sharper edge but don't mind a bit more maintenance. Ceramic blades are another choice—lightweight and corrosion-proof, yet prone to chipping if dropped. Whichever you select, keep it clean by washing with soapy water and drying thoroughly after each session. Using a small amount of isopropyl alcohol can help with sanitisation, even if no blood is involved. Store your knife in a protective sleeve or sheath so it doesn't bump into other objects, as dents or nicks can change how the blade moves on the skin.

. . .

3.7 Transport and Storage: Being Mindful of the Law

Laws surrounding knife possession vary widely. When you need to transport a knife, consider storing it in a locked case or at least keeping it somewhere that isn't immediately accessible, like the boot of a car. A small label or lockable pouch can signal that you're carrying the blade responsibly, minimising potential legal issues. It's always best to look up local regulations, so you know the rules you're expected to follow.

3.8 Preparing Your Scene and Minimising Risks

Even with a perfectly chosen and maintained knife, accidents can happen if you rush into play without any preparation. Before you begin, check the blade for any signs of damage, ensure there's enough room to move without stumbling into objects, and plan where you'll set the knife down if you need a free hand. A designated surface—like a small table or tray—keeps your scene organised and lowers the risk of the knife falling onto the floor or you accidentally grabbing it at a precarious angle.

3.9 Adaptations for Different Abilities and Needs

Not everyone has the same level of grip strength or physical mobility, but that doesn't have to exclude anyone from enjoying knife play. A blade with an ergonomic handle can ease strain on the wrists, while a lighter style of knife may feel more comfortable if you have concerns about joint stability. Some people prefer to stay seated or lie down during scenes, so they don't have to support their full weight while concentrating on blade control. Communication aids —such as hand signals or a discreet buzzer—can also help you stay aware of your partner's feelings if verbal cues become difficult.

3.10 Countering Myths about Knife Choice

It's easy to fall into the trap of thinking that a bigger knife inherently equals a more intense or exciting scene. In truth, size alone doesn't guarantee a satisfying experience. The same is true for the assumption that a single knife style can handle any scenario. Different scenes may call for different blades, and some styles simply won't suit every person's grip or comfort level. Another myth is that plastic knives must be safer, yet a cheaply made one might break unexpectedly, leaving sharp fragments or an unsteady jagged edge. A well-crafted metal blade that's looked after and used with care is often far more reliable.

• • •

3.11 Emotional Resonance and Cultural Perspectives

Knives can carry strong cultural meanings. In some places, they symbolise protection, ceremony, or heritage; in others, they may spark fear or be intertwined with negative experiences. On a personal level, a blade's style can set the mood of a scene, whether you opt for something discreet and minimalist or a design that looks bold and tactical. Discussing any cultural or emotional associations you might have can help ensure everyone involved feels at ease and doesn't encounter surprises that undermine the moment's sense of trust.

3.12 Assembling a Knife Kit

If you see yourself continuing to explore knife play, it can be handy to put together a small kit. This might include your primary knife, a backup blade, cleaning supplies like a soft cloth and alcohol wipes, and a few basic first-aid items such as plasters, bandages and antiseptic cream. Storing it all in a single place— preferably locked or clearly labelled—makes it straightforward to prepare for a scene. It also helps you keep track of what condition your knife is in, so you're not fumbling around at the last minute looking for a safe blade.

3.13 Practising on Your Own: Building Confidence

If you're the person holding the knife, you can boost your confidence by practising simple movements without a partner. Gently tracing the spine or the flat of the blade along your own arm or leg can help you learn how much pressure feels natural and how the knife responds when you change angles. Taking a moment to observe your arm, wrist, and grip in a mirror can also refine your technique. Even small steps like these ensure that when you bring a knife into a partner-based scene, you're less likely to have shaky hands or awkward movements that could break the mood or cause an accidental scratch.

3.14 Conclusion: Integrating the Right Knife into Your Play

A carefully chosen knife, combined with mindful preparation and upkeep, forms the backbone of a satisfying knife-play experience. When you match the right blade to your style—whether that's a small paring knife for subtlety or a more substantial utility knife for a balanced mix of show and control—you set the scene for heightened sensations that remain firmly within the realm of consent and trust. Paying attention to factors like grip, sharpness, and cultural resonance can help you shape scenes that are both exciting and respectful of personal boundaries.

As you move forward, remember that no one knife is perfect for every situation. Feel free to experiment, try out different styles, and develop your own comfort level with handling. With time and practice, you'll discover the kind of blade that truly enhances your scenes, opening up new dimensions of tactile and psychological pleasure—without compromising the safety and well-being of everyone involved.

Next, we'll delve into the body's response to a blade, looking at safe zones, how to read your partner's reactions, and strategies to ensure the experience stays enjoyable on both physical and emotional levels.

Chapter 4

Better Understanding the Human Body

Knife play might look like it's centred on the blade, but there's an equally important dimension: the body beneath it. Knowing where and how to place a knife can dramatically change both the safety and the sensation of a scene. In this chapter, we'll explore the different zones of the body, discuss how various areas respond to external knife play, and consider the personal factors—such as body type, medical conditions, or past experiences—that can shape your approach. When you understand which areas are less risky and which demand extra caution, you'll be better equipped to create scenes that remain thrilling without crossing into harmful territory.

4.1 Why Location Matters

Every time a knife glides over the skin, it makes contact with nerves, blood vessels, and layers of tissue beneath the surface. Even if you're not piercing the skin, too much pressure or a slip in a sensitive spot can lead to unintended pain, bruising, or emotional distress. Having a basic grasp of surface anatomy can help you avoid situations where you're relying on guesswork at a critical moment. Different parts of the body also offer unique balances between sensation and safety. Some regions are fleshy, with fewer vulnerable blood vessels or nerve clusters near the surface, while others sit closer to large arteries or highly sensitive tissues. The goal is to pick areas where a blade can be traced or lightly pressed without endangering your partner.

4.2 Sensation Versus Risk

One of the core decisions you'll make when planning a knife-play scene is how much physical and psychological intensity you want to generate. Safer zones, like the upper arms or shoulders, can still provide a mind-stirring experience, purely because the presence of a knife brings a layer of tension. You don't necessarily have to move into high-risk areas, such as the neck or the inner thigh, to create an impactful scene. However, if you do explore regions that are inherently more vulnerable, please approach them with the utmost caution, especially if major blood vessels lie just beneath the skin. Remember that the line between exciting and unsafe can be thin when you're dealing with sharper, more sensitive zones.

4.3 Understanding Surface Anatomy in Knife Play

For external knife play, you're mostly dealing with the outermost skin layer. The sensation your partner feels comes from stimulating the nerves close to the epidermis, which can be surprisingly responsive to even light pressure. Beneath the skin, there's fat and muscle that you shouldn't be pressing into with a knife, since our aim here is purely surface-level contact. If you're aware of how thin or thick certain areas of skin tend to be, you'll have a better sense of how to adjust your angle and pressure. This knowledge can help you play confidently, minimising the chance of accidental pain or injury.

4.4 Safer Zones for External Play

Certain parts of the body are generally considered less hazardous when it comes to surface contact with a blade. The upper arms and shoulders are good examples because they're well-padded with muscle, which makes accidental harm less likely. They're also sensitive enough to give a clear sense of the metal's coolness or the slight drag of its edge, but not so sensitive that every touch feels overwhelming. The outer thighs offer a similar balance of muscle coverage and responsiveness to changes in temperature or pressure. Many people also find the upper or mid-back to be a workable area, though it's usually less sensitive. The psychological element in a back-focused scene can still be potent, particularly because the person on the receiving end can't always see what's happening behind them. Lastly, the buttocks can be a surprisingly safe choice, thanks to the subcutaneous fat and muscle structure, though consent is key here, as some partners find that zone more intimate than others.

4.5 Proceed with Caution: Riskier Areas

Other parts of the body might be tempting to explore but carry extra layers of risk. The inner thigh, for example, is famously sensitive and erotically charged, yet the femoral artery lies near the surface. If you're drawn to that area, using very light pressure and constantly checking in can help reduce the likelihood of injury, but the risk remains significantly higher than with a shoulder or outer thigh. The lower abdomen can also be a tricky spot due to thinner protective layers and the possibility of past medical issues like surgeries. With the ribcage, the challenge comes from its tendency to provoke involuntary squirms—some people are quite ticklish, which might cause sudden movements. Anywhere movement is unpredictable, your control of the knife needs to be especially precise to prevent mishaps.

. . .

4.6 Strict No-Go Zones without Advanced Training

Certain areas stand out as too dangerous to attempt in casual external play, especially if you're relatively new. The neck and throat hold major arteries and the windpipe, so any miscalculation can become serious very quickly. The face is another region best left alone unless you and your partner are both extremely experienced and comfortable, because facial cuts carry not only physical risks but emotional consequences as well. Meanwhile, the chest area around the nipples contains sensitive tissue and fewer natural protective layers, which can lead to discomfort or unintended damage. It's not that advanced knife players never venture into these zones, but they do so only after thorough training, careful negotiation, and deep mutual trust.

4.7 Individual Variations: Body Type, Medical Concerns, and Trauma

No two bodies are identical, and what one person finds safe might be too intense for someone else. Some people have thicker layers of fat or muscle, which can offer more protection, while others are more slender or have scarring that affects nerve sensitivity. Medical conditions—whether they're related to the skin, blood, or past surgeries—can change how certain body parts respond to pressure. Emotional history also matters. If a partner has trauma tied to a specific region, even a gentle blade in that spot can provoke strong emotional distress. Discussing these factors well before you begin is essential for ensuring the scene goes smoothly.

4.8 Reading Physical and Emotional Responses

Body language is a powerful indicator of how your partner is handling the scene. Tense shoulders, flinching, or a sudden shift in breathing can all be signs of growing discomfort. At times, your partner might lean in or relax, suggesting they want more of what you're doing. Ongoing communication—both verbal and non-verbal—is vital to maintaining a sense of safety. Encourage your partner to speak up if the sensation turns from thrilling to overwhelming, and be open to adjusting your technique or relocating the knife to a different area. Emotional cues are equally important; a sudden wave of anxiety or tearfulness might mean you need to pause and process what's happening before you continue.

4.9 Body Mapping as a Negotiation Tool

One practical way to clarify which areas are in play is through body mapping. Some partners talk through this verbally, while others sketch a simple outline of the body and mark zones as safe, cautious, or off-limits. This can help you negotiate each region's comfort level without confusion. For example, your partner might mark the outer thighs as an enthusiastic "yes," the inner thighs as a "maybe, with light pressure," and the neck as a firm "no." Having this reference can calm nerves on both sides, ensuring you don't wander into a high-risk or emotionally charged area unwittingly.

4.10 Bringing It All Together During a Scene

A knife-play session often works best when you begin in the safer zones. This lets you warm up your partner to the sensation of metal against their skin and gauge their comfort level. If things go well, you can gradually move toward more sensitive or psychologically intense areas, assuming you both agree. The critical point is to keep lines of communication open, so you know if a movement or location is becoming too much. Being prepared to adapt mid-scene—whether that means shifting to a different part of the body or adjusting the angle and pressure—helps keep the experience enjoyable rather than alarming.

4.11 Respecting Individual Limits and Intersectional Factors

People's comfort with knife play can also be influenced by cultural norms, gender identity, and personal or religious beliefs about the body. Certain cultures may consider some body parts taboo, or individuals might experience dysphoria related to particular areas if they're trans or gender non-conforming. Physical disabilities might require modifications, such as seated or angled positions that reduce strain. The key is to recognise that every person's set of boundaries is shaped by a blend of physical, emotional, and societal factors. Having these discussions before you start is crucial for a scene that feels inclusive and respectful.

4.12 Conclusion: Location, Sensation, and Consent

Understanding how different zones of the body respond to knife play is a fundamental step in keeping your scenes safe, consensual, and deeply satisfying. While certain areas, like the upper arms or outer thighs, can often be explored with minimal risk, others demand a higher level of caution and experience. Factoring in body type, medical history, and emotional triggers helps tailor the scene to the individual, ensuring that you're not simply relying on general advice when a more personalised approach might be needed.

Keep an eye on physical and emotional signals, and don't be afraid to pause or shift focus the moment anything seems off. By pairing thorough knowledge of the body with respectful communication, you lay the groundwork for knife play that is as mindful as it is thrilling.

Chapter 5

The Psychology of Knife Play

Knife play is not just about technique—it's about the emotions it creates within you and your partner. Introducing a blade into a play scene can tap into primal reactions such as fear, excitement, and trust. The psychological charge often becomes the main draw, adding a layer of intensity that goes beyond mere physical touch.

In this chapter, we'll explore how knife play can provoke powerful emotions, how to manage those feelings responsibly, and how to balance arousal with genuine safety. We'll also consider the role of trust, vulnerability, and aftercare, making sure you maintain a healthy mental state before, during, and after any scene that involves a blade.

5.1 Why Knives Trigger Strong Reactions

Many of us grow up associating knives with danger or violence, whether from watching films, reading news stories, or simply hearing that they are sharp and potentially lethal. When that same object is introduced into an intimate context, those learned alarm bells can ring loudly, sending adrenaline rushing through your system. Even in a setting of full consent and respect, seeing or feeling a blade near your skin can produce a heady mixture of excitement, trepidation, and heightened awareness.

One major factor is the fear element. A controlled measure of fear can amplify arousal and deepen emotional bonding, provided both partners agree to explore it and remain able to pull back if it becomes overwhelming. In many ways, knife play is a dance between excitement and self-preservation, and mastering that dance relies on both partners' capacity to recognise the point at which "thrilling" starts to become "genuinely frightening." Knives also carry a symbolic weight that can intensify any existing power dynamic. The person wielding the blade may feel an amplified sense of control, while the person on the receiving end may experience a heightened state of vulnerability. This can be erotic in a Dominant/submissive context or simply an additional layer of intensity for those who prefer more sensation-based play. Either way, the emotional responses linked to knives—ranging from an urge to flee to a surprising sense of surrender—are worth considering well before the scene begins.

. . .

5.2 Emotional Preparedness: Setting the Stage

Before you bring a knife into your scene, it's important to reflect on your own emotional and mental readiness. If you're already feeling off-balance due to stress, sadness, or anger, a high-adrenaline activity like knife play may not be the wisest choice that day. Ask yourself whether you're seeking a jolt of excitement to lift your mood or if you're in a stable enough frame of mind to handle the rush of adrenaline that knife play can bring. It's also helpful to clarify what you want out of the experience—are you seeking a suspenseful, fear-based thrill, or a more meditative exploration of sensation?

Emotional boundaries matter just as much as physical ones. You might be fine with the blade tracing along your arms and legs but find the idea of having it near your abdomen too unsettling, especially if you've had surgery there or carry past trauma. Openly discussing these sensitivities—or any limits around how intense the scene can get—allows your partner to navigate the emotional territory with care. Some people prefer a brief conversation, while others find it helpful to use pre-scene checklists or quick verbal affirmations, such as "Are we both in a good headspace to do this today?" or "Is there anything weighing on your mind that I should know about?" These small gestures can build an atmosphere of mutual respect and reassurance from the start.

. . .

5.3 Fear Play versus Sensation Play

Knife play can serve different purposes, and it's worth distinguishing between fear-based and purely sensation-focused approaches. Some people enjoy the rush of fear, skilfully orchestrated to remain within safe bounds. A scene like this might involve hovering the knife close to the skin, introducing sudden movements to make the heart race, or whispering tantalising threats that invoke a sense of danger while never stepping outside the agreed-upon limits. If you're topping in a fear-play scenario, keep a close eye on your partner's breathing patterns, facial expressions, and body language. Checking in verbally —such as asking, "On a scale from one to ten, how intense does this feel?"—can help you gauge whether their enjoyment is holding steady or crossing into genuine distress.

On the other hand, some people prefer to skip the fear factor entirely, relishing the cool brush of steel as a sensual experience. They might find it meditative or grounding, focusing on the smooth glide of the blade or the contrast of metal against warm skin. The knowledge that the knife could cause harm if misused is still presen, but the aim is not to induce fear. Instead, it becomes an exercise in heightened touch and close attention to your partner's response. Recognising these two very different styles of knife play—one powered by fear, the other by pure sensation—can help you and your partner decide on the mood and methods that suit you best.

5.4 Trust is everything

Trust is at the heart of any BDSM activity, and that trust must be particularly solid when knives come into the equation. It often takes time to build this kind of confidence in each other's intentions and abilities. Many partners start cautiously, such as limiting knife contact to one or two areas on the body before expanding as comfort grows. Each positive encounter lays the groundwork for deeper or more experimental scenes, and both partners learn to interpret each other's reactions with greater precision.

Communication can help maintain that trust throughout the scene. Some people use a steady stream of narration—quietly stating where the knife will go next, or offering reassurances such as "You're safe, I'm here, and I have full control." Others prefer to keep talking to a minimum, maintaining a charged silence that deepens the focus. Ultimately, how much or how little you speak depends on what sustains the scene's atmosphere without sacrificing clarity. The crucial part is ensuring that you can both detect any shift in mood or comfort level, even if you're not constantly chatting.

· · ·

5.5 The Body's Chemical Responses: Adrenaline and Endorphins

One of the most fascinating aspects of knife play is how your body can react chemically. An adrenaline surge might sharpen your senses, heighten your emotional responses, and temporarily mask mild discomfort. This can feel exhilarating, creating a blend of excitement and even euphoria, but it does carry a caveat: once the scene ends, the body may experience an "endorphin crash." Some people feel unsteady, low, or extra emotional hours or days after an intense encounter. It's completely normal to have these ups and downs. Planning your aftercare— whether that means cuddling, quiet rest, or simply staying in touch to talk through how you're feeling— helps smooth out the transition back to everyday life.

5.6 Case Study: Balancing Fear and Comfort

Consider a couple who want to explore a playful yet edgy scene. One partner enjoys mild fear and the psychological charge of the blade's proximity, while the other partner is keen but worried about accidentally going too far. They decide to begin with a short session, using a small, relatively dull knife and avoiding riskier body areas. Throughout the scene, the bottom rates their level of intensity on a simple numeric scale—anything above seven signals that it's time to slow down or pause for a quick check-in. By the time they reach the end of the scene, both partners find that the blend of anticipation, trust, and careful technique delivers the exact balance of thrill and safety they were hoping for.

5.7 Final Thoughts

Knife play can be a potent mixture of fear, adrenaline, intimacy, and connection. If you decide to incorporate it into your BDSM practice, taking the time to define whether you're seeking a fear-based thrill or a purely sensual experience will shape how you conduct the scene. Building trust gradually—through gentle, short sessions and consistent communication—gives both partners a sturdy foundation to explore more intense variations later on. It also prepares you to handle the emotional highs and lows that can arise, ensuring that any powerful feelings are processed rather than left to linger in confusion.

Most importantly, know that boundaries, communication, and aftercare are every bit as crucial in knife play as the blade itself. By respecting each other's comfort levels and remaining alert to shifts in mood or mental state, you can explore the captivating edge of knife play with confidence. In the next chapter, we'll turn our attention to how you might structure a scene overall—deciding how to set the atmosphere, integrate knife play with other elements of BDSM, and guide your partner through a memorable experience without straying into unintended harm.

Chapter 6

Power Dynamics & Sensory Play

When people hear about knife play, it's easy to imagine a scenario where a dominant figure looms over a vulnerable partner, brandishing a blade to emphasise control. While those scenes certainly exist within BDSM, they're just one possibility in a wide spectrum.

Knife play can also be entirely sensory, focusing on the glide of metal across skin, without invoking any form of power exchange.

This chapter looks at the different roles people can take on—whether as a top, bottom, switch, or power bottom—and highlights how the interplay of power can range from explicit and hierarchical to fully equal. We'll also discuss how holding the blade does not necessarily mean holding all the power, and why the concept of "power" in BDSM can be more fluid than many realise.

. . .

6.1 Power Dynamics: A Quick Refresher

In the broader context of BDSM, the Dominant (often referred to as Dom or Domme) typically sets the tone of a scene, deciding on its pace and level of intensity, though always within previously negotiated limits. The submissive (or sub) agrees to relinquish a measure of control, trusting the Dominant to lead them through the experience. This arrangement, however, is not as rigid as it might appear from the outside, and each partnership adapts these labels in its own way. A Dominant could be stern or nurturing, while a submissive might be playful, bratty, or quietly obedient.

When knife play enters the picture, it often involves one partner wielding the blade and the other receiving its sensations. The psychological charge of seeing someone hold a knife can reinforce the sense of one person guiding the activity while the other places trust in their hands. Yet knife play doesn't always require a fixed Dominant/submissive framework. Some people prefer to switch roles periodically, while others embrace a flat, egalitarian approach with no power differential at all. Knife play can be wrapped in intense fear play or simply enjoyed for the sensation of cool steel on skin.

6.2 Purely Sensory Exchanges

A common misunderstanding is that knife play must be anchored in a clear power hierarchy, but that isn't necessarily the case. Two partners may be equally curious about the feeling of a blade and decide to explore it together without any aura of dominance or submission. In this sort of scene, they might take turns tracing a dull knife across each other's arms, backs, or thighs, simply to experience the tingling sensation of metal against skin. This approach can be akin to a gentle massage, except with the added novelty of a blade.

Sensory-based knife play appeals to those who love experimenting with different textures or temperatures but aren't interested in psychological tension. The focus remains on bodily reactions and shared curiosity rather than on who is in control. Communication still plays an essential role—both people need to stay aware of any discomfort or anxiety that might arise when metal meets skin—but the energy in this style of play is more cooperative than hierarchical.

6.3 Common Roles in Knife Play Scenes

Although many assume that the person holding the knife must be the Dominant, the reality is more nuanced. The top, who typically applies the blade, can lead in a very directive way—telling the bottom exactly how to position themselves, perhaps adding a strong element of control and intimidation if that's what both partners desire. Alternatively, the top could act more like a service provider, responding to the bottom's guidance on where and how to move the blade, creating a scene that centres on the bottom's comfort and preferences.

For the bottom, receiving the blade's touch might be a submissive act of trusting the top not to harm them. Yet some bottoms prefer to remain more active, directing the top about where to place the blade and how much pressure feels right, which can blur the lines between who is truly "in charge." Switches, meanwhile, can embrace both perspectives, potentially shifting roles in different scenes or even halfway through the same one. This flexibility might add an extra layer of adventure, as each partner experiences being both the knife-wielder and the one feeling the knife's touch.

6.4 Power Bottoming and 'Bottoming from the Top'

The term "power bottom" describes a person who is on the receiving end of sensation but still holds a significant amount of influence over how the scene unfolds. If a bottom wants the blade to stay on their upper thighs and not venture near their abdomen, they might give real-time instructions to the top. They may specify how much pressure they want, request a quicker or slower pace, or even shape the emotional atmosphere by indicating whether they want whispered reassurances or an air of dramatic suspense. This approach allows the bottom to remain physically vulnerable while steering the overall direction, balancing surrender with an element of command.

"Bottoming from the top" is a similar dynamic, where the individual theoretically in the submissive role issues consistent directives to the supposed Dominant. Sometimes this is the intended style, creating a playful inversion of roles. At other times, it happens unintentionally, causing confusion or tension if the scene was initially meant to be top-led. Having a conversation about how much input the bottom can —and should—provide keeps everyone on the same page. It's perfectly valid to want a structured power-exchange scene where the top guides every step, just as it's valid to prefer a back-and-forth collaboration where the bottom's voice is always prominent.

6.5 What Power Dynamics Bring to Knife Play

Whether strict or relaxed, any power dynamic can heighten the psychological impact of knife play. Introducing a knife already raises the stakes, as both partners must stay fully focused on safety. If one person wields the blade and the other is instructed not to move, the tension and thrill can shoot up quickly, especially if there's an element of fear or suspense woven into the scene. This type of setup often relies heavily on trust: the bottom needs to feel confident that, despite appearances, the top has their well-being firmly in mind. Meanwhile, the top shoulders the responsibility of controlling the blade's angle and maintaining constant awareness of the bottom's reactions. The intensity can draw partners closer, forging a deeply memorable encounter underpinned by mutual respect.

6.6 Structuring a Knife Scene Without Power Exchange

For those who prefer a more equal footing, an "all-sensory" approach can be equally rewarding. In such scenes, participants might discuss boundaries and techniques beforehand but dispense with the notion of one person "in charge." They could stand or lie side by side, taking turns to explore each other's skin with the knife's flat edge, the dull spine, or a gentle, angled tip. The dialogue tends to be quite open and relaxed, more akin to "How does this feel?" than "Don't move until I say so." Even without a formal power structure, clear communication remains vital: both partners need a safe word or a gesture that indicates if anything feels too intense, painful, or emotionally distressing.

6.7 Negotiating Roles and Limits Before a Knife Scene

Before you introduce a blade into your play, it's wise to talk through what you want to gain from the experience. Is the scene designed to be a show of dominance, with the bottom told to remain perfectly still and comply with every instruction? Or is it a shared exploration, with both of you on an equal footing? Sorting out these questions ahead of time helps you avoid misunderstandings mid-scene, particularly if you're experimenting with knife play for the first time. You should also cover details such as safe words or signals—especially in any fear-based scenario—so that either partner can indicate discomfort or a need to slow down.

Emotional safety is just as important as physical safety in a scene that can feel edgy or taboo. Checking in with each other before, during, and after ensures that no one is carrying anxiety they'd rather not voice. This is especially true in scenes where a strong power dynamic is at play and the bottom might feel vulnerable acknowledging discomfort.

6.8 Wrapping Up: Finding Your Comfort Zone with Roles

Knife play naturally amps up the intensity of a BDSM scene, but the specific roles and power structures you choose can vary immensely. Some pairs crave the electric charge of a Dominant/submissive dynamic with the knife as a potent symbol of control, while others prefer a more equal, sensory-oriented exploration of metal against skin. It's also common for partners to experiment with different styles over time, switching roles or adjusting how overt the power dynamic feels from one scene to the next.

What matters most is maintaining clear communication, explicit consent, and a commitment to safety—both emotional and physical. When you're dealing with something as potentially risky as a blade, a strong foundation of trust and understanding can turn knife play into a thrilling, intimate, and profoundly respectful experience.

Chapter 7
Trauma-Aware Kink Play

Even with meticulous planning and a commitment to mutual respect, the heightened intensity of knife play can bring up powerful emotional reactions— sometimes in the moment, sometimes long after the scene ends. People come to knife play with a wide variety of personal histories, mental health backgrounds, and coping mechanisms, all of which can influence how they process fear and intimacy involving a blade. In this chapter, we'll delve into trauma-informed approaches to knife play, discussing how to recognise potential triggers, manage emotional overwhelm, and ensure that aftercare thoroughly addresses both physical and emotional needs.

7.1 Why Trauma Awareness Matters in Knife Play

The Emotional Weight of a Blade

Knives carry a strong cultural and personal symbolism. They can be seen as tools of violence or aggression, yet they can also represent protection and empowerment. Even if a person has no prior history of being threatened with a knife, the presence of a blade in an intimate setting might trigger anxiety, flashbacks, or an adrenaline surge. Recognising this possibility allows both partners to be prepared for the unexpected. Trauma doesn't always follow a predictable path, so having a plan to handle emotional surges is a vital aspect of safe and nurturing play.

More Than Just Physical Safety

Although earlier chapters have explained ways to avoid cuts and maintain control, emotional well-being is just as critical. Trauma does not show up on the surface in the same way a physical wound might; it can be inward, manifesting as sudden panic or dissociation. Because knife play taps into some of our most primal fear responses, emotional harm can linger if it isn't dealt with sensitively. It's important to remember that encountering trauma-related distress is not a failure of planning—it's an opportunity to respond with empathy and understanding.

Shared Responsibility in Trauma-Informed Play

If you're the one holding the knife, you're also guiding a deeply psychological experience. You don't have to be a mental health professional to be trauma-aware, but you do need a willingness to listen closely, watch out for signs of distress, and be ready to pause or de-escalate the scene if needed. This sense of shared responsibility in knife play nurtures trust, reinforcing a more caring and empathetic BDSM community.

7.2 Recognising Trauma Triggers

Common Trauma Triggers in Knife Play

Any number of past experiences can influence how a person reacts to the feel or sight of a blade. Some might have survived violence involving a knife, while others may have trauma from medical procedures that left them anxious around sharp instruments. Even without specific knife-related experiences, general PTSD or anxiety can heighten someone's stress responses during play. Understanding that these triggers exist, and being open to the idea that they may surface unexpectedly, encourages a supportive and informed approach.

Signs of a Triggered Response

If someone becomes triggered, the signs can range from rapid breathing, racing heartbeat, and an intense desire to flee, to going silent, appearing detached, or breaking into tears. Identifying these behaviours early is essential to prevent the situation from escalating. If you notice any shift in demeanour —such as panic or sudden freezing—pause right away and take steps to reassure, ground, or comfort your partner. Quick intervention can often prevent prolonged distress or emotional harm.

Trauma-Informed Pre-Scene Check-Ins

A simple conversation before knife play begins can make all the difference. Asking, "Have you ever felt threatened by a knife before?" or "Is there anything that might unexpectedly trigger you?" allows your partner to disclose as much or as little as they feel comfortable sharing. They may suggest safer alternatives for where to focus the blade, or mention techniques—like slow breathing or gentle physical reassurance—that help them feel grounded if anxiety arises. Encouraging open dialogue without forcing anyone to disclose painful details builds trust and sets the tone for a safer, more compassionate scene.

7.3 Strategies for Minimising Trauma Responses

Grounding and Slow Escalation

Some participants benefit from gradually acclimatising to the presence of a knife. This could mean showing them the blade in a neutral setting first, letting them hold it or observe how you handle it before any actual play begins. When you do make contact, start with the spine of the knife, keeping pressure low and movements deliberate. Ask simple check-in questions—"How does this feel? Are you comfortable?"—rather than relying solely on a safe word. These steps help create a sense of control and reduce the risk of emotional shock.

Titration: Introducing Sensation in Small Doses

Titration is a psychological approach that involves gradually exposing someone to a stimulus, giving them the opportunity to adjust at each step. In knife play, this might mean first allowing your partner to watch as you trace the flat side of the blade along your own arm. When they seem comfortable, you move on to lightly touching the spine of the blade to a "safer" area on their body. Only when trust is firmly established might you move towards more intense zones, such as the inner thighs or near the throat. This process lets both partners monitor emotional and physical responses, making it easier to step back or adjust if something feels too intense.

7.4 Managing Emotional Overwhelm During a Scene

Immediate Steps If a Trigger Happens

If you notice your partner slipping into distress—whether it's panic, dissociation, or an urgent need to escape—stop or slow down immediately. Put the knife aside somewhere safe, try to orient them with calm statements such as "You're safe" or "I'm here," and gauge whether they need gentle touch or would prefer more space. Modelling slow, steady breathing can help them refocus, and changing the environment—turning on lights or playing calming music—can signal that the scene's tone is shifting. If none of these measures settle their distress, it's best to end the scene entirely and move into aftercare.

When to End a Scene

The moment it's clear that the bottom's distress is not subsiding, or is escalating, the right choice is to conclude the scene. Aftercare then becomes the priority. Your partner's emotional and mental wellbeing should always overshadow the desire to continue any form of play, however intense or fulfilling it may be.

7.5 Deep Dive into Emotional Aftercare

Why Aftercare Is Essential

Knife play can lead to adrenaline highs, which often come with emotional crashes once the excitement fades. This crash might appear as sadness, anxiety, irritability, or a feeling of emptiness that sets in hours —or even days—later. Providing strong aftercare helps cushion this drop. After a scene that stirs powerful feelings of fear, arousal, or trust, a calm and comforting period of recovery can make all the difference in leaving your partner feeling safe rather than emotionally raw.

Components of Effective Aftercare

Physical comfort—such as blankets, warm drinks, or a gentle massage—can ground your partner in the here and now. Open-ended conversations about how each of you experienced the scene also support emotional processing. Some people benefit from a type of grounding where they hold a familiar object or focus on the physical sensations of breathing slowly. It's wise to check in again over the following day or two because sometimes emotional aftershocks don't surface immediately. Being available for a quick chat or text exchange can reassure your partner that you're still there to support them.

7.6 Final Thoughts on Trauma Awareness and Emotional Safety

Knife play goes beyond mere technique or the thrill of danger. It's an intimate, psychologically charged act that can unlock deep fears or emotional responses, particularly if a partner carries hidden or not-so-hidden trauma. Approaching these scenes with empathy and a readiness to adapt ensures that the excitement remains centred on mutual pleasure and growth, rather than causing harm. Prevention strategies like slow acclimation, regular check-ins, and careful escalation help keep both participants emotionally regulated. And if distress does occur, pausing the scene or ending it altogether underscores the value you place on your partner's emotional wellbeing.

Ultimately, trauma-informed knife play respects that each person's past can shape how they react to a blade in the present. By integrating compassion, thorough communication, and sensitive aftercare, you create a space where the intensity of knife play can be explored without risking emotional harm—a space where connection and trust have the freedom to deepen, even as the edge of the blade comes into contact with the surface of the skin.

Chapter 8

Crafting the Scene

After learning about safety measures, knife selection, anatomical considerations, and the psychology of this kink, you may be wondering how to combine these elements into a coherent, satisfying scene. This chapter aims to guide you through that process, from your initial discussions to the final moments of aftercare. By mapping out a scene in advance, you can focus on shared pleasure and connection rather than second-guessing each step.

8.1 Negotiation: The Foundation of a Scene

Even if you have some experience in BDSM, a detailed negotiation is particularly important with knife play. Thorough, open dialogue reduces the likelihood of misunderstandings or unintentional harm, especially if you're experimenting with a technique or style that's new to one or both partners.

Whether you prefer a casual conversation or a more structured approach, the goal is for everyone involved to feel knowledgeable and prepared.

Start by stating your goals. Is the scene intended to be playful, lightly erotic, or does it involve some controlled fear? Next, clarify any limits, including which body parts are absolutely off-limits and which might be acceptable with caution. Even if you have a familiar safe word from previous scenes, confirm it again and agree on any non-verbal signals you might need. Decide on which knives you'll be using, how sharp they are, and roughly how long you'd like the scene to last. Lastly, spend some time discussing what aftercare might look like. By finishing this conversation with a shared plan, you'll give yourselves the best possible starting point.

8.2 Creating the Right Environment

The physical setting can greatly influence how a knife-play scene unfolds. Privacy is often a top concern; interruption mid-scene can jar both partners out of the mood and compromise safety. If you enjoy a certain ambience—whether that's low lighting for an intimate feel or clear visibility to keep an eye on the blade—set this up in advance. Music can also help shape the atmosphere, adding tension or serenity, depending on your preferences.

When it comes to furniture, think about stability and practicality. A sofa or bed might be too soft if you're aiming for controlled movements, whereas a sturdy table or a comfortable mat on the floor may offer better support. Keep a small "safety station" within easy reach, with items like towels, first-aid supplies, and anything else you might need in a pinch.

8.3 Scene Flow and Pacing

A successful knife-play scene often unfolds in stages, beginning with a gentle warm-up and building to a peak of intensity before winding down. You might start by making verbal contact: a simple question such as, "Are you feeling comfortable and ready to begin?" can affirm your partner's mindset. Following this, a grounding touch—a light hand on the shoulder or a brief massage—helps establish trust before the blade ever comes into view. Once the knife is introduced, let your partner see it and perhaps hear it tapping lightly on a surface to stimulate anticipation.

From there, you can gradually increase the intensity by moving to new body areas or varying how the blade is applied—tracing the spine, pressing the flat edge, or combining it with other sensations if you've agreed to incorporate additional elements. Keep a close watch on how your partner reacts. If they tense up or go quiet, pause and ask if they're still happy to continue. This kind of steady communication ensures you're both engaged and allows you to adapt the experience in real time.

8.4 Techniques for External-Only Knife Play

Although knife play revolves around the presence of a blade, there are numerous ways to explore without breaking the skin. Try alternating between the dull spine and the flat side of the knife, creating contrasting sensations. Some enjoy gliding a chilled blade across warm skin to heighten the stark difference in temperature. Others prefer focusing on precise, gentle tip play in areas that are less risky, confining the blade to fleshy zones rather than venturing toward sensitive spots.

Another way to enhance the scene is by changing your partner's sensory input. Placing a blindfold over their eyes can sharpen their awareness of each slight touch or shift in angle. Alternatively, you might make deliberate use of verbal cues to build suspense, describing what you're about to do or making them wait for contact until they're practically holding their breath.

8.5 Communication Throughout the Scene

Even if you've mapped out the scene thoroughly, things can change in the moment. You or your partner could suddenly feel an unexpected wave of apprehension or excitement. Maintaining clear communication is crucial. Simple check-ins like "Is this pressure okay?" or "Would you like more of that?" can go a long way in keeping both people aligned. If anyone is unable to speak, use established non-verbal signs—a tap on the surface, a squeeze of the hand, or something else that clearly indicates a need to slow down or pause.

Being attuned to body language is just as important as verbal dialogue. A partner who leans into the knife might be signalling enjoyment, whereas someone who goes rigid might be teetering on the edge of discomfort. Responding promptly to these cues helps sustain the trust that underpins knife play.

8.6 Aftercare: Guiding the Descent

The climax of a knife-play scene can be intense, and it's important to guide your partner back to emotional equilibrium once it's over. Some people find physical warmth—like a blanket or simple embrace—calms and reassures them. Others need a few moments of quiet, perhaps accompanied by water or a snack if the adrenaline rush has left them feeling drained. You could also choose to talk through what happened, sharing the highlights and clarifying any uncertainties while the experience is still fresh.

Remember that emotional aftershocks can appear much later, so a follow-up text or call the next day can offer reassurance. It can also provide a chance to discuss what you both enjoyed, what you might change next time, and whether you'd like to explore further or try something new.

8.7 Putting It All Together: A Sample Scenario

Imagine someone who is new to knife play but eager to experience the tension of a blade. After a thorough negotiation, you set the stage by dimming the lights and placing a first-aid kit discreetly in the corner. Your partner lies down on a stable surface, and you begin with a gentle touch on their shoulder, checking in to ensure they feel calm. Once they confirm they're ready, you bring out the knife, letting them see and hear it before lightly running the spine across a less sensitive area, like their upper arm. As they become more comfortable, you expand to other spots, building up to the peak when you press the flat of the blade against a more sensitive place, heightening the suspense. When you sense your partner's breathing quicken or their body tense, you slow back down, eventually putting the knife aside as a clear signal that the scene is reaching its end. The two of you share quiet time afterward, exchanging impressions of what worked best and ensuring any lingering adrenaline fades into a sense of safety and trust.

8.8 Conclusion: The Art of Scene Crafting

Designing a knife-play scene is a creative endeavour that blends careful negotiation, thoughtful preparation, and active communication. From the moment you start planning until the final wave of aftercare, each step matters. A well-structured scene not only mitigates risk but also amplifies the excitement and connection between you and your partner. By pacing the action thoughtfully, staying attentive to verbal and non-verbal signals, and ending on a note of mutual reassurance, you ensure that knife play becomes a memorable and deeply satisfying experience for everyone involved.

Chapter 9

Blending Knife Play with Other Kinks

Knife play already brings a distinctive blend of psychological charge and tactile contrast, yet many find it even more engaging when combined with other kinks. Whether your interest lies in bondage, temperature shifts, roleplay, or impact play, the integration of additional elements can introduce fresh dimensions to your scenes. In this chapter, we'll explore how to merge these practices without compromising the defining thrill of a blade in action.

9.1 The Appeal of Combining Knife Play with Other Kinks

A major draw of multi-kink scenes is the way they deepen and diversify sensation. The cold press of steel can feel even more pronounced if the body has just been warmed by wax or if a partner is restrained, unable to flinch away. This layered approach also allows for shifts in emotional tone over the course of a single session. You might begin with a calm, exploratory mood—slowly drifting into tension and suspense once the knife is introduced—only to bring the energy back down with a gentler activity. These variations help keep participants engaged and prevent the experience from becoming too predictable.

In addition, combining multiple kinks can be practical. If your available time for play is limited, weaving various elements together can give the session a sense of momentum. Rather than setting aside separate "mini-scenes" for each activity, everything flows as one cohesive narrative.

9.2 Managing Complexity in Multi-Kink Scenes

However exhilarating it might be to incorporate several activities, doing so requires extra attention to detail. If you plan to tie a partner's hands or feet, make sure the restraint doesn't interfere with safe knife handling. Placing a blindfold over their eyes can heighten their senses, yet it also removes visual feedback that might otherwise signal discomfort or danger. Likewise, if you're adding impact play, keep track of where all implements are at any given moment—nothing disrupts a scene faster than fumbling for the correct tool or accidentally using the wrong one.

For the person wielding the blade, multi-tasking becomes a central skill. You could be monitoring rope tension, adjusting the temperature of a chilled blade, tracking your partner's reactions, and upholding any role-play scripts you've set in place. Staying calm and organised helps maintain the intensity without overwhelming yourself or your partner. Meanwhile, from the receiver's perspective, the sudden variety of sensations can be both enthralling and disorienting. Check-ins become especially vital, as it's easy for someone to become overstimulated if too many stimuli are layered in quick succession.

9.3 Popular Pairings: Where Knife Play Thrives

Bondage and Restraint

Incorporating restraint magnifies the knife's psychological impact, as the inability to move away underscores the vulnerability aspect. Some enjoy a slow, deliberate method—perhaps wrapping a partner in layers of plastic or cloth before artfully slicing them free. Others find a beautiful tension in tying someone to a piece of furniture and casually running the blade across exposed areas. Whichever approach you choose, practise cutting (for example, rope) on spare materials beforehand so you're confident in your technique.

Sensory Deprivation

Taking away one or more senses can make the introduction of a blade incredibly intense. A partner with their eyes covered might jump at even the gentlest contact, uncertain when and where the next touch will come. Adding headphones or other forms of sound muffling can heighten this effect even more. The suspense and disorientation become a key part of the scene, so be prepared to communicate through other means if someone seems overwhelmed.

Roleplay Scenarios

Knives often carry connotations of power and danger, which can be harnessed in a variety of roleplay plots—ranging from stylised interrogation scenes to mythical or ritualistic narratives. By weaving the knife into the story, you infuse it with more than just physical significance. The act of tracing symbols on someone's skin or pressing the blade lightly against their throat can feel like stepping into a vivid, shared fantasy.

Temperature Contrasts

Metal is an excellent conductor of temperature, allowing you to shift quickly between extremes. A chilled knife pressed suddenly to warm skin can prompt a sharp intake of breath, and re-warming the blade (or the partner's body) just as swiftly can create a cycle of alternating tension and relief. Some find it effective to pair these temperature fluctuations with roleplay or bondage elements, orchestrating a scene that continuously challenges the receiver's senses.

Impact Play

The rhythmic pattern of flogging, spanking, or paddling creates a kind of comforting predictability—until you pause that routine to introduce the knife's chill. The abrupt change in sensation can be a jarring yet exhilarating twist. Alternatively, you might hold a small paddle in one hand and the knife in the other, switching between different types of contact in a way that keeps your partner on edge (both literally and metaphorically).

9.4 Troubleshooting Multi-Kink Knife Play

Combining kinks opens the door to unique experiences, yet it can also lead to confusion or strain if not handled with care. Planning a loose sequence ahead of time—bondage first, knife play second, short break, then perhaps a brief roleplay—gives the scene structure without rigidly scripting every moment. During the scene, subtle check-ins help keep you informed about your partner's physical and emotional state. Even a softly whispered "Are you still with me?" can make all the difference in maintaining that delicate balance between excitement and overload.

If things become overwhelming at any point—too many sensations, or a sense that the partner receiving them can't fully process what's happening—it's perfectly acceptable to scale back. Pausing a particular activity or switching focus to simpler forms of touch can provide a breather, allowing the scene to continue rather than grinding to an uncomfortable halt.

9.5 When Simplicity May Be Best

While multi-kink combinations can be thrilling, some sessions might benefit from a narrower focus on knife play alone. This can be especially helpful if you're new to using a blade in BDSM contexts or if you prefer exploring the nuances of one activity at a time. Streamlining your scene doesn't make it less intense; it can actually deepen your understanding of knife play by removing distractions. The absence of ropes, blindfolds, or other props lets both partners devote their full attention to the sensations and psychological aspects connected to the blade.

9.6 Final Thoughts: Exploring Multi-Kink Creativity

For many, the excitement of knife play lies partly in its adaptability. The same blade that provides a subtle, spine-tingling caress in one scenario can become an adrenaline-laced focal point in another. By merging knife play with different kinks, you open up countless possibilities, each with its own emotional tone and physical intensity. The trick is knowing your limits and your partner's comfort zone, then layering new elements in a way that heightens—rather than overwhelms—the unique dynamic that knife play brings.

If you've mastered the fundamentals of blade handling and established strong lines of communication, the next step is to let your creativity take the lead. Whether you're adding a gentle shimmer of wax, orchestrating a dramatic interrogation roleplay, or testing a partner's senses with surprise touches, there's no shortage of ways to shape multi-kink scenes that feel cohesive, daring, and deeply rewarding.

Chapter 10

Skill-Building & Exercises

Developing confidence in knife play requires more than simply reading or discussing techniques. True skill emerges through consistent, hands-on practice that refines your physical control and hones your emotional awareness. This chapter offers a series of exercises and drills designed to guide both tops and bottoms towards safer, more intuitive experiences. We'll also consider how to structure practice sessions, whether you're working solo or with a partner, so that every step of your journey becomes an opportunity to deepen trust and competence.

10.1 Why Practice Matters

Reading about knife play or listening to others' experiences provides useful background, but there is no substitute for feeling a blade against a surface in real time. As the top, you need to know how much pressure is required to move the knife smoothly without cutting, and how to hold it at various angles. Deliberate repetition helps your grip become steady rather than tentative. When your own movements feel reliable, the person beneath your blade can relax more fully, confident that you won't slip or exert too much force.

For the partner receiving the knife's touch, practice is equally important. You might discover early on that certain areas of your body are more responsive than expected, or that you need to distinguish a pleasant rush of adrenaline from a warning sign of genuine distress. By becoming familiar with your own reactions, you can communicate more effectively with the top during an actual scene, facilitating a safer, more enjoyable encounter.

10.2 Setting Up a Practice Space

Before you begin any drill, it helps to establish a stable, calm environment. If you're practising alone, choose a spot like a kitchen counter or a sturdy table where you can test your knife-handling techniques without clutter or distractions. Keeping your phone within reach but silenced ensures you're not caught off-guard by emergencies or notifications.

When you're working with a partner, make the space reflect the care you'd put into a real scene. A private area where neither of you will be interrupted is ideal.

Some people prefer a casual, chatty atmosphere during practice, whereas others replicate the focused energy they'd use in an actual BDSM setting. Either approach is valid, as long as both participants remain attentive.

10.3 Foundational Drills for the Top

Confidence behind the blade can grow from simple, repetitive exercises. For instance, you could use a piece of fruit on a cutting board to gauge how lightly you can rest the tip without breaking the surface. This kind of exercise reveals how little pressure is needed to puncture or slice, clarifying the margin of error you have when working with human skin.

Another useful drill involves practising broad, sweeping arcs across a cushion or pillow, holding the knife at different angles to understand how the blade's orientation affects friction. Varying between the knife's spine and its flat side also helps you get comfortable switching sensations mid-movement. Finally, you might consider adding hand-strength or grip workouts to your routine. Squeezing stress balls, rotating your wrists with light weights, or performing controlled lifts can alleviate fatigue and trembling during prolonged knife play sessions.

10.4 Exercises for the Bottom's Comfort and Self-Awareness

Equally important are drills that help the receiver learn how their body responds. One straightforward method is self-tracing with a blunt or dull blade, typically on the arm or leg. Try to notice if a certain angle provokes immediate anxiety or if you feel more apprehension when you bring the knife closer to a sensitive spot. Deep, rhythmic breathing can serve as an anchor, reminding you that you remain in control of your emotional state.

Practising with a mirror can also be illuminating. Have your partner run the dull side of the knife along visible areas while you watch how your body reacts. If you notice your shoulders tensing or your expression tightening, this is a chance to verbalise what you're feeling—perhaps a mixture of thrill and unease—helping you develop a better vocabulary for future scenes.

10.5 Partnered Drills for Coordinated Confidence

When two people practise together, it's crucial that each person can stop or redirect the action at any moment. One exercise involves the top gliding the knife across a willing partner's skin while the partner periodically calls out "Stop." Upon hearing this, the top must freeze instantly, demonstrating attentiveness and control. Such pauses give the bottom a way to test how quickly their partner responds and fosters mutual trust.

Another approach is to role-play safe words in a low-stakes setting. The receiver can occasionally say "Red," prompting the top to halt all movement, or "Yellow," signalling a need to ease off. Even if there's no discomfort yet, this habit of immediate response ensures both partners remain comfortable with the idea that the scene can be paused or ended at any time.

10.6 Building Emotional Resilience During Practice

Physical drills alone won't eliminate performance jitters if you haven't also practised staying centred under stress. Techniques like deep breathing, visualisation, or repeating affirmations—such as "I'm capable and focused"—can help calm nerves. For the receiving partner, gradual exposure is often helpful. Start by observing the knife at a distance, then allow gentle contact on a safe area of the body, proceeding to more intense touches only when you feel ready.

It's also wise to debrief after each session. Discuss what felt smooth and confident, which parts triggered anxiety, and how you might adapt next time. A single positive experience can act as a strong anchor, reassuring both participants that they can handle more advanced manoeuvres later.

10.7 Turning Practice into Progress

To keep advancing, try setting small goals for each session. You might aim to maintain a perfectly steady grip for a whole minute or practise switching angles without lifting the blade awkwardly. Tracking your progress in a journal or note-taking app can motivate you to keep improving. If you reach a point where the basic drills become second nature, consider experimenting with new exercises—perhaps trying a slightly sharper knife, or adding simple roleplay elements to simulate a real scene.

Rewarding yourself when you hit a milestone—such as acquiring a new blade that you've had your eye on or planning a more elaborate scene to put your refined skills into practice—can keep the journey enjoyable. Over time, you'll likely notice that your self-assurance in knife play translates into a calmer, more self-possessed demeanour during actual scenes.

10.8 Final Thoughts: Mastery Through Repetition

Practising knife play is less about seeking perfection than it is about building familiarity and confidence. By steadily honing your technique and learning to interpret your own emotional cues (as well as your partner's), you equip yourself for satisfying, well-orchestrated scenes. Drills tailored to tops help combat shaky hands and uncertain grips, while exercises for bottoms encourage greater self-awareness and communication. Partnered sessions allow you both to synchronise your cues, ensuring an immediate response to any shift in comfort level.

Like most BDSM skills, knife play becomes more natural through patient repetition and a willingness to reflect on each step. The next chapter addresses common misunderstandings, handles frequently asked questions, and suggests ways to navigate concerns from peers or partners. As you integrate practical exercises with clear, ongoing communication, you'll find yourself increasingly prepared to explore knife play with skill, poise, and a well-earned sense of trust.

Chapter 11
Debunking Myths & FAQ

Even within BDSM circles, knife play can spark confusion or be portrayed in overly dramatic ways. Some assume it must involve blood, while others believe it's only for those who seek extreme danger or pain. In truth, as you've discovered, knife play can be a measured, non-penetrative form of kink that centres on trust, sensory exploration, and psychological tension. This chapter clarifies some widespread misunderstandings and answers common questions, enabling you to approach knife play with greater confidence and awareness.

11.1 Myth-Busting: Common Misconceptions

Myth One: Knife Play Always Involves Blood or Cutting

The belief that knife play requires drawing blood often stems from more extreme practices, yet what we've discussed so far involves only external, non-penetrative contact. The coolness of steel, the controlled pressure, and the subtle edge of fear can be achieved without puncturing skin. While some do venture into forms that involve cutting, that's a distinct branch of play that calls for advanced skills and precautions.

Myth Two: It's Only for Hardcore Thrill-Seekers

Another misconception is that you must crave intense fear or high levels of pain to enjoy knife play. In reality, many people engage with blades in a gentle, playful manner, finding the thrill in anticipation or in the careful dance of sensation. This practice needn't be terrifying or extreme; it can be sensual, teasing, and even soothing if approached with the right mindset.

Myth Three: Knife Play Cannot Be Safe

While there are always risks when introducing a sharp object into a scene, stating that knife play is inherently unsafe overlooks how preparation and communication can greatly reduce hazards. Clear negotiation, proper technique, and ongoing check-ins can render non-penetrative knife play as controlled as many other forms of BDSM. Safety lies in informed choices and respect for limits, rather than in banning a particular implement outright.

Myth Four: A Dull Blade Is Always Safer

It might seem logical that a dull blade would pose fewer dangers, but a poorly sharpened knife can slip more easily, increasing the risk of accidental injury. A moderately sharp blade, handled with care, generally requires less force and allows for more precision. Skill and caution matter more than the blade's sharpness alone.

Myth Five: It's Strictly a Dom/sub Activity

While knife play often appears in power exchange contexts, it can also be practised in entirely equal settings. Partners may take turns exploring the tactile qualities of a blade on each other's skin without emphasising hierarchy. Alternatively, solo participants might experiment with careful self-application of the blade's spine or flat side. The dynamics are flexible, determined by the players' preferences rather than a fixed set of rules.

Myth Six: If You're Not Afraid, You're Doing It Wrong

Some assume that fear is the primary goal of knife play. Although certain individuals do enjoy ramping up the tension, others prefer mild, intriguing sensations without any element of dread. The beauty of knife play lies in its adaptability—it can be as adrenaline-charged or as soothingly hypnotic as you and your partner choose to make it.

11.2 Frequently Asked Questions

Q: What if I'm worried about the sight of blood?

There's no need for blood to enter the picture at all. Non-penetrative techniques focus on the cool feel of metal and the psychological edge of having a blade nearby. If you dislike even the idea of a sharp edge, start with the dull spine or a less pointed tool, easing into the concept gradually.

Q: How do I stop myself from panicking about hurting someone?

It's normal to worry about causing harm. To combat this anxiety, practise alone first by running a blade along soft objects like fruit or cushions. When you introduce it to your partner, do so slowly, sticking to low-risk areas. Honest communication will reassure both of you, and each positive experience will boost your confidence.

Q: Is it possible to manage knife play if I have shaky hands?

Yes, though you may need extra caution and more frequent breaks. A blade with a comfortable grip and a manageable size can help. Focus on deliberate, measured movements rather than rapid ones, and let your partner know about any coordination challenges so they can offer clear feedback if the pressure becomes uneasy.

Q: Does knife play always have to be dark and serious?

Not at all. While some enjoy an intense, dramatic vibe, others keep it light-hearted or erotic without any heavy themes. A playful approach—perhaps involving banter or gentle teasing—can be just as engaging as a high-tension scene. The tone is yours to set.

Q: Should I consider wearing gloves during knife play?

Gloves can improve grip if your hands are prone to sweating or you're dealing with a particularly slick handle. However, they may diminish your tactile awareness. If you opt for gloves, experiment beforehand to ensure you can still gauge pressure effectively.

Q: How do I bring up knife play with a partner who's never tried it?

Approach the subject calmly and openly, explaining what interests you about it—whether it's the sensation of metal, the element of trust, or the psychological tension. Reassure them that you only wish to explore external contact and are happy to proceed slowly, respecting their comfort and boundaries.

Q: What if my partner has a history of trauma involving knives?

In that case, proceed with caution or accept that they may never want to engage. Trauma is complex, and no kink is more important than your partner's emotional safety. If they're curious but anxious, take micro-steps —starting with the visual presence of a blade or gentle contact in a safe area, always pausing at the first sign of distress.

Q: Are there legal restrictions on owning or carrying certain knives for play?

Local laws vary greatly, so do a bit of research to avoid any potential issues. Some places ban specific blade lengths or types, while others regulate how knives can be transported. Staying informed keeps you on the right side of the law.

Q: What if I accidentally draw blood during non-penetrative play?

If you do nick the skin, stop immediately and switch to first-aid mode. Clean the area, dress any wound if necessary, and check on your partner's comfort. You may choose to end the scene there, depending on how severe or unsettling the accident is, and use the experience to identify what went wrong for future reference.

Q: Is solo knife play an option?

Yes, though additional caution is required. You'll want to ensure you have a stable surface, good lighting, and a plan for dealing with any slips. Some people enjoy the thrill of self-applied sensation, but it's vital to avoid areas you can't see clearly or control with steady hands.

· · ·

11.3 Final Thoughts: Dispelling Fear with Knowledge

Misconceptions about knife play often stem from exaggerated depictions or confusion about what "edge play" really entails. By recognising that blades can be used without cutting and that the aim might be gentle tension rather than outright terror, you open up a realm of possibilities that emphasise trust, communication, and carefully managed risk. Clear information and hands-on practice help demystify the process, transforming what might look intimidating into a controlled, collaborative experience.

Chapter 12

Elevating Your
Knife Play

After building a solid foundation—understanding blades, honing basic control, and experimenting with psychological cues—you may be ready to take your knife play to a more sophisticated level. At this stage, the emphasis shifts towards refining your technique, integrating layered psychological elements, and weaving multi-faceted scenes that challenge both mind and body. This chapter explores advanced methods intended to deepen your practice, ensuring each moment carries a sense of precision, creativity, and mutual trust.

12.1 Refining Blade Handling: Advanced Physical Techniques

By this point, your grip and angle control should feel instinctive rather than forced. Now is the time to broaden your range of motions and consider how subtle shifts in pressure, speed, or temperature can raise the intensity. One advanced approach is the feathering technique, where you move the flat of the blade with barely-there contact across the skin. The objective is to produce a lightly ticklish, yet undeniably charged sensation, creating a continuous wave of awareness without startling the receiver.

On the opposite end of the spectrum, you might explore a more deliberate style known as the pressure trace. Here, you guide the blade's edge or tip in a slow, unwavering line, applying a measured weight that leaves the recipient hyper-focused on the exact trajectory. This method thrives on disciplined micro-adjustments—tiny increments of added or reduced force that can produce a world of difference in how the sensation is perceived.

Another option involves incorporating brief, staccato-like touches that alternate with moments of stillness. In these instances, use short, controlled taps of either the spine or the sharpened edge, then pause just as swiftly, so your partner remains on high alert for what might follow next. If you feel fully comfortable with single-blade work, you may try dual-knife play. Holding two knives simultaneously—using one for gentle tracing and the other for sharper, more pronounced contact—heightens complexity, demanding a deep level of concentration to coordinate both hands.

．．．

12.2 Advanced Psychological Layers

Beyond physical prowess, many find that the true appeal of advanced knife play lies in the subtle but potent mental and emotional dimensions it can invoke. If you're drawn to themes of power exchange, you can underscore that dynamic by letting the blade become an extension of your authority in the scene, whether you choose to keep it near at all times or bring it into play only after building up suspense. The mere sight of a blade hovering just out of reach can elevate the tension, prompting your partner's breath to catch as they wait for that first cool contact.

Some scenes delve even deeper into emotional catharsis. In these situations, the process of carefully applying the knife, combined with the intangible thrill it provides, can help the person receiving it experience a sense of release. This might manifest as a shedding of stress or a moment of heightened vulnerability, where the act of being so intimately touched by something inherently dangerous sparks an intense emotional response. Planning a thorough debrief or extended aftercare becomes especially important if you suspect such a depth of feeling may arise.

12.3 Integrating Knife Play into Extended Scenes

Expanding the timeframe allows for a more layered exploration of knife play. A longer session might begin with gentle, almost playful strokes that serve as a warm-up, gradually introducing periods of heightened tension where you adopt sharper angles or heavier pressure. You might then scale back, focusing on lighter, teasing passes again to let the anticipation build. Eventually, you can push towards a peak moment of concentrated intensity, before smoothly bringing the energy back down.

Some prefer to add extra elements that complement knife play, such as shifting the partner's body position, introducing varied textures, or employing different forms of sensory distraction. For instance, switching between a chilled blade and a warm hand can create quick shocks of contrast. Alternatively, you might combine auditory cues—whispering instructions or counting out each slow pass of the blade—to keep your partner grounded in the moment. These tactics draw attention to each movement, preventing the scene from becoming monotonous and helping both participants remain vividly engaged.

12.4 Negotiated Weapon Play for Experienced Partners

When you've reached a point of unwavering trust, you might consider weaving the knife more integrally into a power-driven framework. This could mean establishing the blade as a symbol of negotiated threat—deciding in advance which parts of the body it can touch, how close it may come to especially vulnerable areas, and what emotional reactions are sought. The art lies in balancing the appearance of danger with the continual reassurance that no actual harm will occur. Repeated, quiet reminders that you're fully in control, and that you care for your partner's safety, can reinforce the intensity of the scene without tipping it into genuine panic.

This approach should be navigated only when both people feel comfortable with more pronounced psychological stakes. If you do so, remain constantly attuned to subtle shifts in mood or body language, and be prepared to adjust or end the segment if anxiety crosses into distress. The thrill of advanced power dynamics in knife play rests on the knowledge that each boundary, no matter how edgy, is still guarded by clear communication and trust.

12.5 Mastering Advanced Knife Play

Ultimately, advancing your knife play revolves around exploring the knife's capacity to induce both tactile and emotional peaks. You may be perfecting complex moves—tracing dual lines, pacing staccato strokes, or applying intense, sustained pressure—while also refining your partner's psychological journey through carefully orchestrated suspense or role-based interplay. The key is never to lose sight of mutual respect and safety, even when chasing the adrenaline that knife play can provide.

Remember that mastery is a continuous journey rather than a fixed endpoint. Each new approach you integrate, whether it's layering multiple sensations or experimenting with drawn-out power exchanges, offers insights into your personal style and limits. Keep communicating with your partner before, during, and after each scene, and regularly assess whether your advanced techniques still align with the trust you've established. By doing so, you'll maintain the delicate equilibrium between excitement and security, ensuring that your progression into more intricate forms of knife play remains a source of genuine connection and exhilaration.

Chapter 13

Learning & Sharing in Community

Although knife play often feels like a private affair shared solely between you and your partner, there can be significant benefits to stepping into a wider network of people who share your curiosity. Engaging with others—whether online or at in-person events—provides fresh perspectives, boosts confidence, and fosters a sense of belonging that can make all the difference in your development. In this chapter, we'll look at ways to find these supportive spaces, what to anticipate from workshops and events, how to recognise reliable mentors, and the importance of sharing your own experiences in a responsible manner.

13.1 Why Community Matters

One of the most valuable aspects of a community is the opportunity to witness a variety of approaches to knife play. Despite all the reading and practice in the world, your experiences are inevitably shaped by personal biases and preferences. Observing someone who frames knife play as a gentle, sensual activity can be enlightening if you've only considered it through the lens of more intense power exchange, and vice versa. Exposure to such diversity helps you refine your sense of what resonates for you.

Community participation also offers real-time critique that no book or article can fully replace. During a workshop, for instance, an experienced practitioner might notice you hold the knife at an odd angle or press too hard on a sensitive area. Their immediate, hands-on feedback can accelerate your learning and help you dodge entrenched bad habits. Additionally, connecting with others who have navigated the emotional and psychological aspects of knife play can offer a sense of relief and normalcy—hearing that your mix of excitement and apprehension is far from unusual can lift a significant mental weight.

13.2 Types of Community Spaces

Various kink-oriented events cater to different comfort levels, so it's worth exploring which environment aligns best with your personality and needs. For a low-pressure introduction, you might start with munches, which are casual gatherings in public venues like cafés or pubs. They give you the chance to meet others in a relaxed setting—

particularly helpful if you find the idea of play parties or dungeon events too daunting at first.

Workshops and skill-sharing gatherings are the next step if you'd like structured guidance. These sessions are usually led by educators who demonstrate techniques and allow participants to try them under supervision. Some instructors rely on demonstration models, letting you observe the precise knife angles and contact methods covered in this guide. Others encourage active participation if you bring your own blade. Meanwhile, play parties and dungeons offer a more immersive atmosphere, where you can witness live scenes—provided you have the hosts' permission and the performers' consent. Watching how people negotiate, signal comfort levels, and maintain safety protocols in real time can be invaluable.

Online forums and social media groups have also become major hubs of information. You'll find an array of platforms that cater to a broad spectrum of BDSM interests, including dedicated sections for edge play. Although it's easy to connect globally, be cautious about accepting every piece of advice at face value—there's no guarantee of expertise in an anonymous post. Prioritise discussions led by knowledgeable users or moderated by experienced admins, and cross-reference what you learn with multiple sources whenever possible.

13.3 Vetting Mentors and Peer Educators

In a community setting, it's not uncommon to encounter individuals who describe themselves as highly experienced in edge play or who offer mentorship. That said, not everyone who claims expertise has genuinely refined their techniques or upholds strong ethical standards. Assessing a potential mentor involves paying attention to how they emphasise safety, remain open to your questions, and respect your emotional comfort. If someone dismisses your concerns, refuses to discuss boundaries, or insists there's only one "correct" way to approach knife play, that's a red flag.

Conversely, good mentors are often upfront about the scope of their experience, encourage you to learn from various sources, and welcome discussions around limits and risk reduction. Asking a few trusted community members about a teacher's reputation can also offer clues about whether they foster a respectful learning environment. Attending one of their workshops or observing them in a public demonstration before you accept one-on-one guidance can give you a chance to see their methods firsthand, helping you decide if they align with your own values.

13.4 Sharing Knowledge Responsibly

Once you've reached a certain level of comfort and skill, you may feel inspired to pass your insights on to others. Doing so can enrich the community and help new people explore knife play with clarity. If you choose to teach, be transparent about how you developed your practice and what aspects you're still exploring. Focusing on safety fundamentals—like careful negotiation, steady technique, and active consent—ensures that newcomers build a strong base rather than being dazzled by flashy moves they aren't yet prepared to manage.

It's also important to avoid gatekeeping. Although guidelines for risk management are necessary, proclaiming that there's only one valid approach to knife play can alienate those who prefer alternative styles or who experience satisfaction in different ways. When giving public demonstrations, make consent paramount for any partner who's modelling with you, and be aware of the venue's rules around edge play—some spaces have stricter boundaries on anything perceived as a weapon. Always keep the learning objective in sight; shock value or stunt-driven theatrics can overshadow actual education and encourage reckless experimentation among impressionable viewers.

13.5 Wrapping Up: Community as a Lifelong Resource

Being part of a kink community—either online, in local gatherings, or both—can considerably enhance your knife play journey. Exposure to diverse methods sharpens your comprehension of what knife play can encompass, while regular feedback helps you sidestep complacency and continue fine-tuning your abilities. For those who thrive in group settings, the collective support and camaraderie can provide a lasting sense of belonging. If you're more private, the option of maintaining anonymity by using a scene name or sticking to quiet observation ensures you can dip your toes in without compromising your comfort.

Ultimately, community is an ongoing source of inspiration, guidance, and sometimes, reality checks—particularly for those times when you need reassurance or advice on how to move forward. By immersing yourself in respectful, well-informed spaces, you grant yourself continuous opportunities to learn, adapt, and flourish in your approach to knife play.

Chapter 14

Continuing the Journey

You've come a long way. From honing fundamental skills to exploring the deeper emotional and psychological dimensions of knife play, you now possess a set of tools—both practical and theoretical —that can guide you through almost any scene. Yet a guide can only take you so far; the real growth lies in blending these principles with your own evolving desires, emotional states, and interpersonal dynamics.

This chapter focuses on how to keep your knife play experiences engaging and meaningful over the long haul. We'll delve into strategies for refining your abilities, strengthening the emotional bonds that arise in these scenes, and approaching your practices with a reflective mindset. You'll also find reminders about safety, boundaries, and your ethical obligations to both yourself and any partners—ensuring that as you push the edges of your exploration, you remain securely grounded.

14.1 Embracing an Evolving Practice

14.1.1 There's No "End Goal"

It's tempting to ask, "When do I become an expert in knife play?" or "How will I know I've reached the finish line?" But in truth, there is no finish line. Even those with years of experience discover fresh angles, techniques, or desires as they continue. Your approach to knife play might shift alongside your personal growth, emotional changes, and the different relationships you form over time. Treat your knife play journey as a perpetual work-in-progress rather than a skill to be mastered once and for all.

14.1.2 Personal Growth Through Kink

Although it's often seen as a standalone kink, knife play can serve as a powerful avenue for personal development. Handling a blade near your partner's skin (or having it near your own) demands openness, honesty, and a willingness to confront fear. These skills—trust, assertive communication, and self-awareness—can bleed into the rest of your life, bolstering your confidence in everyday settings. When you learn to hold your ground in a scene, you might discover that you're also more poised about drawing boundaries elsewhere or voicing your needs in personal or professional situations.

14.1.3 Revisiting and Revising Limits

We often assume that boundaries, once set, remain static. Yet what thrilled you initially may feel routine a year later, and a limit that once seemed unthinkable might gradually spark your interest. It's wise to reassess your limits periodically. Ask yourself whether certain techniques still excite you or whether a new scenario appeals. Equally, be alert to circumstances where you might need to slow down or pull back. Knife play should continue to bring satisfaction and growth, not feel like an obligation driven by your past self.

14.2 Strengthening Emotional Intimacy and Trust

14.2.1 Communication That Deepens Over Time

Knife play hinges on mutual vulnerability and the willingness to communicate openly. While you may have developed a good rapport with your partner, never assume you fully grasp their internal state. Stress, health changes, and shifts in relationship dynamics can all influence how someone experiences a blade. Regularly checking in—both verbally and through non-verbal cues—keeps each scene aligned with current emotional realities.

14.2.2 Balancing Spontaneity and Structure

Because the idea of a knife near the skin can be both electrifying and unsettling, some find it reassuring to plan each scene meticulously, while others prefer a more spontaneous approach. Finding a balance can be as simple as using a code like "Yellow" or "Red" to quickly flag when you need to pause or stop. This fluidity supports moments of natural escalation without sacrificing the safety net of clear communication.

14.2.3 Evolving Aftercare Rituals

Just as your style of knife play matures, your aftercare needs may also evolve. In the early stages, you might require substantial reassurance or physical comfort after an intense experience. Later, you might crave something more low-key—perhaps joking around, sharing a meal, or taking a quiet walk. Being open to adjusting your aftercare ensures that you and your partner remain genuinely soothed and connected once the blades are put away.

14.3 Lifelong Learning and Community Engagement

14.3.1 Advanced Workshops and Peer Exchanges

Even if you're already confident handling a knife, advanced-level workshops can reveal finer details of grip, angle, or scene pacing you may not have encountered before. If your local community doesn't offer such events, consider organising one. Sharing techniques with peers provides an energising environment for everyone involved.

14.3.2 Exploring Other Kinks

Knife play blends seamlessly with a range of BDSM practices. You could incorporate rope bondage to heighten a partner's sense of helplessness or intersperse the blade with impact play for bursts of contrasting sensations. Wax play, too, can amplify every stroke of the knife if you apply warm wax and follow it up with the cool edge of steel. Approaching scenes with a broad skill set helps keep them fresh, nuanced, and collaborative.

14.3.3 Knowledge Outside BDSM Circles

There's no need to limit your exploration purely to kink-oriented resources. Learning about wrist control or grip strength from martial arts, understanding cutting angles from culinary training, or diving into psychological research about fear can all enhance your intuitive sense of what makes knife play work. This cross-disciplinary awareness often adds depth to your scenes and increases your overall confidence.

14.4 Self-Reflection and Ethical Growth

14.4.1 Journaling and Debriefing

Maintaining a simple log or journal can be hugely beneficial. By noting what felt natural, what felt off, and how you responded emotionally, you create a record of your development. Over time, patterns emerge—perhaps you'll see that you thrive on prolonged, slow-building tension, or that quick bursts of intensity fit you better. Periodically rereading these observations can help clarify future directions and steer you away from repeated missteps.

14.4.2 Trusting Your Intuition

As your competence grows, you'll increasingly rely on non-verbal cues and an internal sense of timing or pressure adjustments. Sometimes this "gut feeling" can defy explanation—maybe you sense your partner tensing before they verbally indicate discomfort. Honouring these intuitive nudges often enhances safety and deepens the emotional resonance of the scene, even if you can't articulate exactly why you chose to ease off at that moment.

14.4.3 Emotional Processing Between Scenes

Some knife play experiences linger, leaving you with a heady mix of exhilaration and introspection. If you encounter scenes that trigger a deeper reaction—whether it's pure delight or a sense of vulnerability—make time to process. Talk openly with your partner if they're also involved, or seek out friends or professionals familiar with kink culture if the emotions feel too layered to handle alone. Ensuring you understand and integrate these feelings paves the way for continued healthy play.

14.5 Final Thoughts: Continuing Your Journey

Knife play isn't just about technique; it's about the profound interplay of trust, sensation, and symbolic meaning that arises when a blade makes contact with skin. As you move forward, keep in mind the foundational values of consensual, risk-aware exploration. Make space for ongoing learning, whether that's pushing your tactile boundaries, experimenting with new scene dynamics, or simply refining your communication skills.

Key Reminders:

• Consent and safety form the bedrock of every encounter.

• Growth is incremental and never truly finished.

• Psychological depth can be as integral as physical skill.

• Community connections and consistent self-reflection nourish your continuing development.

• Boundaries and emotional well-being must always take precedence over ambition or curiosity.

Where you go next is up to you. Perhaps you'll refine your knife-handling precision further, experiment with multi-sensory experiences, or mentor newcomers keen to learn. Whichever path you take, let curiosity, mindfulness, and respect guide you. With these principles as your compass, you can cultivate knife play scenarios that bring a blend of thrill, trust, and intimacy well into the future.

About the Author

Sarah is a qualified Counsellor and Social Worker. In 2020, she founded Progressive Therapeutic Collective, a sex-positive and kink-affirming mental health practice.

She lives on Dja Dja Wurrung land in Australia, where sovereignty was never ceded.

Kink, power dynamics, and sensory play are areas Sarah is deeply passionate about—both personally and professionally. Her work focuses on building safer and better-informed play communities.

This book is just the beginning of a broader conversation on edge play. It's an invitation to explore kink in a thoughtful, informed, and responsible way.

🖸

www.ingramcontent.com/pod-product-compliance
Lightning Source LLC
Chambersburg PA
CBHW060509280326
41933CB00014B/2903